the little book of

yoga

First published in Great Britain in 2025 by Godsfield, an imprint of
Octopus Publishing Group Ltd
Carmelite House
50 Victoria Embankment
London EC4Y 0DZ
www.octopusbooks.co.uk

An Hachette UK Company
www.hachette.co.uk

The authorised representative in the EEA is Hachette Ireland,
8 Castlecourt Centre, Castleknock Road,
Castleknock, Dublin 15, D15 YF6A, Ireland

Copyright © Octopus Publishing Group Limited 2025

Distributed in the US by Hachette Book Group
1290 Avenue of the Americas, 4th and 5th Floors
New York, NY 10104

Distributed in Canada by Canadian Manda Group
664 Annette St.
Toronto, Ontario, Canada M6S 2C8

All rights reserved. No part of this work may be reproduced or utilized in any
form or by any means, electronic or mechanical, including photocopying,
recording or by any information storage and retrieval system, without the prior
written permission of the publisher.

Lisa Hood has asserted her right under the Copyright, Designs and Patents Act
1988 to be identified as the author of this work.

ISBN 978 1 8418 1593 0

A CIP catalogue record for this book is available from the British Library.

Printed and bound in China

10 9 8 7 6 5 4 3 2 1

Publisher: Lucy Pessell
Editor: Feyi Oyesanya
Designer: Isobel Platt
Assistant Editor: Samina Rahman
Production Controller: Allison Gonsalves
Illustrations: Basae

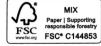

the little book of

yoga

How to perfect 50 asanas & build your own flows

Lisa Hood

GODSFIELD

About
the author

Lisa is a yoga and ritual space holder,
and author. Her company LAHoodyoga is
an in-person and online community that offers
empowering creative yoga sequences and deep
healing rituals and ceremonies. Her practices
infuse the moon phases, crystals, the plant
medicine cacao, tarot and oracle readings
with yang movement and yin stillness.

Lisa strives to create easy, accessible time for
her community to bridge the gap between body,
mind and heart and present opportunities for
people to connect with themselves and believe
the power that they hold within.
@lahoodyoga

Contents

Introduction

Yoga is an ancient practice for the body and mind. Rooted in Indian philosophy, it began as a spiritual practice, and for thousands of years it has hooked practitioners as a way of promoting physical and mental wellbeing with a focus on breathing, flexibility and strength.

Modern yoga is most strongly associated with the physical practice of asana – a series of postures often weaved together in styles such as Vinyasa flows or Ashtanga. Asana practice is generally intended to build strength and stamina, to improve flexibility, coordination, and balance, and to relax the body. However, this provides only one small aspect of the tradition of yoga as a whole.

Yoga is a personal journey, and the beauty of it is that you don't have to be a yogi to reap the benefits. No matter who you are, yoga has the power to calm the mind, strengthen the body, and improve your flexibility and posture. Don't be

intimidated
by yoga
terminology,
fancy studios and
complicated poses –
yoga is for everyone.

When we practise yoga, we are
physically moving energy around
our body; blood will pump, you get a
little warm, you release endorphins
and hormones that create this all-
over feel-good sensation in the body
and mind. Rolling out your mat
ready for practice is an affirmation
that you want to devote time to
yourself. It is a great act of love
toward yourself, and, from that,
it becomes deeply healing.

We can use yoga to release and
surrender, so that we can move
forward into a more balanced,
clear-headed, and harmonious
way of life.

How To Use This Book

The intention of this book is to empower you to practice yoga in your own way, create your own sequences and have fun with it. Yoga can be practised anywhere, and provided that you tune into your body and mind, and you don't push too far, easing yourself in gently, you can explore yoga and all its benefits without needing to attend classes. All you need is a yoga mat and some soft loose clothing, plus a bolster and two yoga bricks if you have them. If not, you could use a couple of pillows wrapped in a towel as a bolster and two large books in place of blocks. Allow yourself to be a guide, let go of all expectations and ease yourself in.

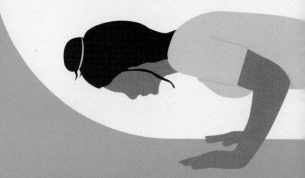

I encourage you to be playful with
your practice and explore new flows and
transitions. Know that some will work, and
others will not, but that's ok. Enjoy the journey.

There are no rules but I do have some suggestions
as to how this book might work for you.

There are six categories of poses:
Warm Up, Warrior, Standing Balance, Seated,
Backbend and Closing. There are also three
Transition categories which act as links and
will help you to move between the poses.

The quickest way to create a flow is to choose
one pose from each of the categories. Grab your
mat, note them down and begin moving the body
through the different poses. Work intuitively, there
is no rush, and see if you can create a
sequence with all the poses you
have chosen.

Creating Flows

Creating flows can be a great way to play with poses, try new things and explore what works for you. Make a list of your selection and try combining the poses in one order, then swap them around and try something new. If you find a sequence that feels great, make a note of the poses so that you can return to it another day.

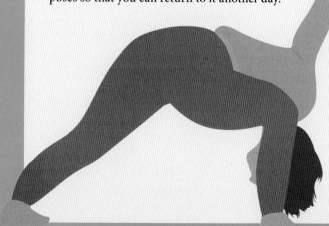

Choosing a position from each category is a quick and easy place to start, but if you have a little more time on your hands (about 20–30 minutes) and would like to create a longer flow, then I would suggest choosing:

2 x Warm Up poses

5 x Warrior poses

2 x Standing Balance poses

2 x Seated poses

3 x Closing poses

2 x Transition poses

Again, this is about being playful. You might want to club together some poses before you start, or just have the book out in front of you as a gentle guide.

On the following pages I've put together three example flows for specific moments in the day. These are a great place to start as a guide, before building your own sequences for a totally personal and unique practice.

Remember to be carefree; this is your yoga and your body, so if you end up doing something completely different then that's ok too!

Transitions

Let's talk about transitions, as these are key in building your flows.

Transitions act like little pathways that guide you in and out of each pose. Sometimes it could be a breath that leads, or maybe it's a step forward, or a lift of the arms. In your self-practice, and when working with this book, your intention should be to move with ease and not feel stuck. If you really tune into your body, feel how you move and try to release any worry about what something looks like, then you can start to make your own transitions. To start with this might feel a little clunky, but in time it will feel easier and become natural, smoother and more grounded.

The most traditional way to transition through a flow is to take a vinyasa.

A vinyasa sequence usually comprises
of the following poses: plank, low plank,
upward dog and downward dog.

If you are new to yoga this can be intense and
quite tiring, so a softer option would be to use only
downward dog as a transition pose. You would make
your selection of poses, and after gently moving
into and holding each pose, take a downward dog,
allowing this to act as a reset and to prepare you for
the next pose. Downward dog can also be used as
a great place from which to take a child's pose, to
find a rest or a breather. As you progress you can
adjust your transition to include other poses,
such as upward dog and low plank, linking
them together as you feel more comfortable.

However you decide to transition
between the poses, think light, think
balanced and be playful. Remember,
if you fall over, it really doesn't
matter! Take a breath and when
you're ready, come back into
the pose.

A Morning Flow

A short and juicy yoga flow in the morning
wakes up the body and mind better than a
cup of coffee – it boosts your heart rate and
endorphins so you can start the day feeling
strong and focused ready for whatever is ahead.
This sequence will take you about 10 minutes.
Try holding each pose for 5 breaths at your
own pace, and don't forget to do both sides!

1. Cat/Cow
2. Downward Dog
3. High Lunge
4. Warrior III
5. Twisted Lunge
6. Plank Pose
7. Twisted Downward Dog
8. Standing Side Stretch
9. Tree Pose

A Bedtime Flow

Bedtime yoga is slow, soft and the perfect antidote to a busy chaotic day. Allow yourself to sink into each pose, and if you can take 8–10 breaths in each one, allowing your body to really melt. This gentle flow will take around 15–20 minutes, and if you are feeling like it's difficult to relax perhaps try placing a towel or blanket on top of your mat, encouraging a softer sensation under the body to help you unwind.

1. Reclined Butterfly
2. Supine Twist
3. Child's Pose
4. Standing Forward Fold
5. Pigeon Pose
6. Sphinx Pose
7. Happy Baby
8. Savasana

The Full Body Practice

For that precious time when you get to spend 30 minutes on your mat, to stretch out and strengthen your entire body. This flow is perfect for any time of day, morning, lunchtime evening. Hold each pose for 3–5 breaths, and if it's your evening practice give yourself an extra-long savasana to really relax the body.

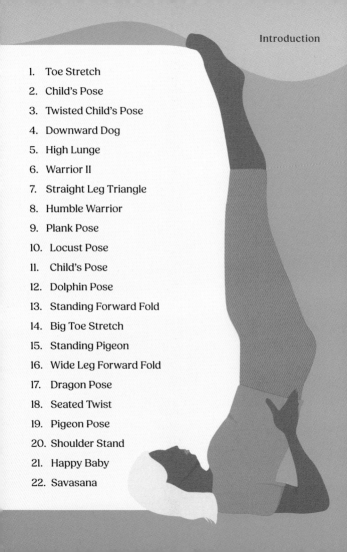

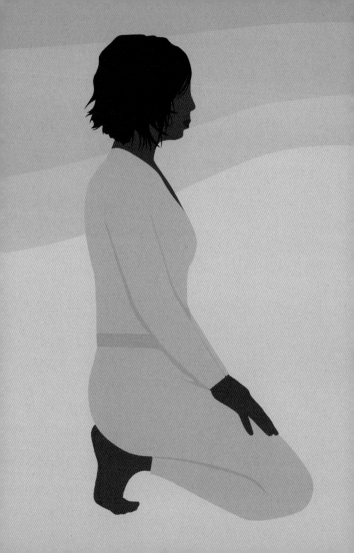

warming poses

Cat-Cow

Marjaryasana-Bitilasana

This is a great warm up pose to do at the beginning of your practice to get the spine moving.

Gently arch and round the back to strengthen and stretch the spine and neck. Connect your breath to the movement to really bring the body and mind together. Inhale as you allow your belly to drop and raise the head, and exhale as you round your spine into cat pose.

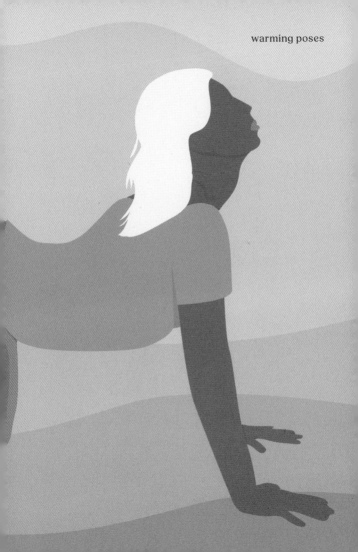

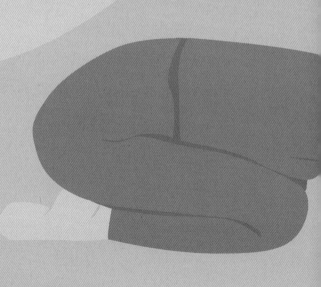

Child's Pose

Balasana

Child's pose is like your best friend in all of your yoga practices. Take this rest pose whenever you need, knees as wide as you like, arms either extended or by your side.

When in this shape you are sending blood flow to your head for focus and clarity, and stretching the lower spine to relieve aches and pains.

Spine Balancing

Utthita Marjaryasana

A core strengthener, this pose is all about elongating your spine. Start on all fours. Think about reaching your arm and leg away from each other as you stretch each one outwards, connecting to your deep inner core.

A pose to improve your focus and concentration, a moment to find your inner strength and power.

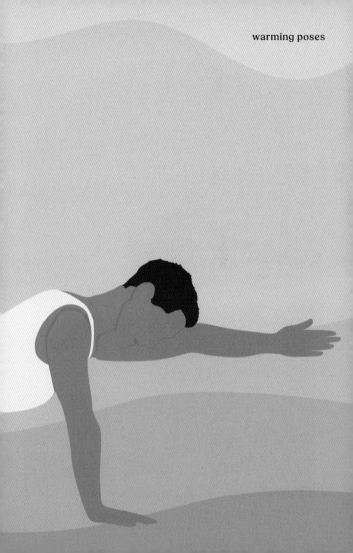

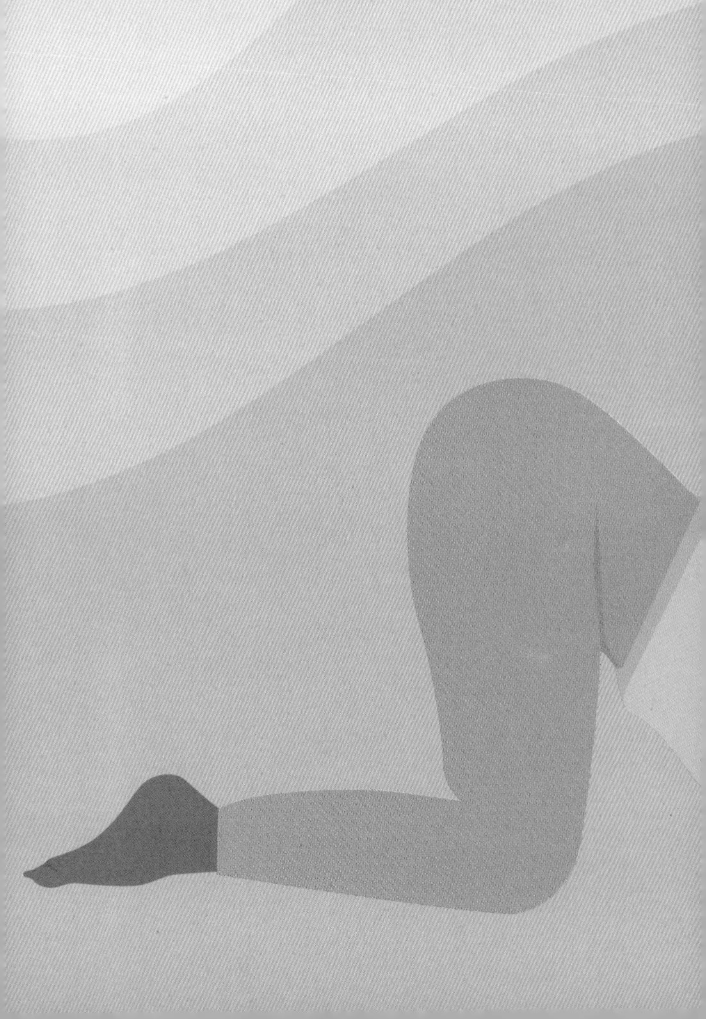

Twisted Child's Pose

Parivrtta Balasana

A wonderful variation of a beautiful resting pose, this combines a forward fold and a twist, allowing the body to unwind itself. Begin in Child's Pose, then thread one arm underneath the opposite side of the body. Repeat on both sides.

Deep twists aid your digestion, and also expand the chest and sides of the torso, allowing your breath to become deep and long.

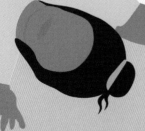

Toe Stretch

Vajrasana

Feeling groggy from waking? Feeling sluggish in the middle of the day? This toe stretch is like having a shot of coffee, a serious pick me up! It enlivens you from the inside out.

Ease into this stretch. Start in a kneeling position, bring the hands to the floor, shift your weight forward and tuck the toes under. Gently bring your bodyweight back onto the toes. Keep your hands on the ground for support at first if needed.

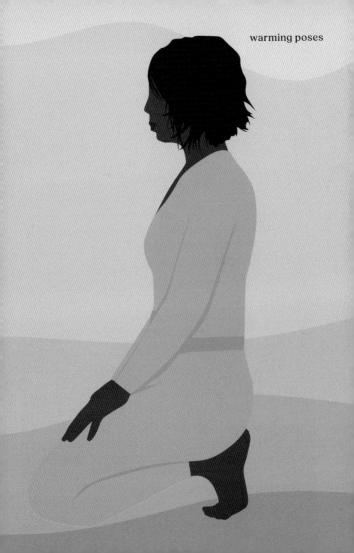

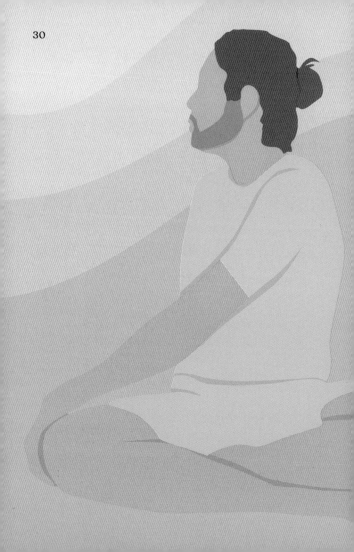

Simple Seated Twist

Parivrtta Sukhasana

The perfect reset for your spine, especially if you've been sat at a desk all day. This seated twist helps to alleviate upper back and neck pain, boosts energy and improves your concentration.

With your legs crossed, place one hand behind your body, the opposite hand onto the other knee, and twist gently, looking over your shoulder. Repeat this on each side for a full reset.

Standing Side Stretch

Parsva Urdhva Hastasana

The juiciest of all juicy
side stretches!

Start standing, hands above the
head, and lean to the left, clasping
the right hand in the left. Allow
the space in between the ribs to
expand, lengthen your breath
and find that beautiful stretch
right at the very top of the hip.
Repeat on the opposite side.

This will improve the
flexibility of your spine and
can aid great posture.

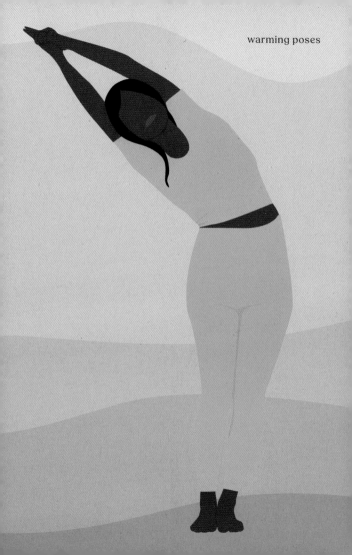

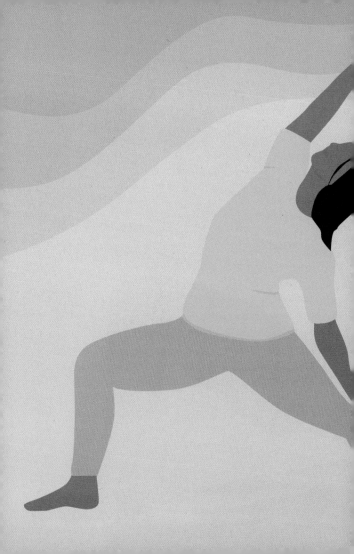

warrior

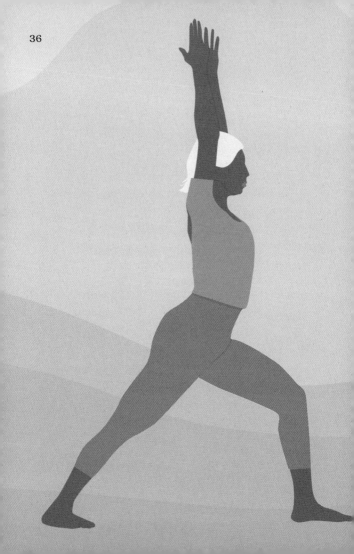

Warrior I

Virabhadrasana I

Warrior I is a foundational standing pose
that uses strength, balance and focus.

When coming into this pose, make sure
your feet aren't directly behind each other;
you should have about half a meter of space
between your feet. You want the energy
of this pose to be forwards and upwards.

It's a challenging pose for both the
body and the mind, promoting good
posture and spinal alignment.

Warrior II

Virabhadrasana II

There is so much strength, power and poise in Warrior II. Your feet should be wide, front foot faces forward and back foot faces more towards the edge of your mat, on a little diagonal. Arms reach out wide like wings, gaze looks towards and beyond your front hand.

Imagine the most beautiful scene in front of you, breeze on your face, sun on your skin, breathing deeply. A pose to remind you to be more warrior than worrier!

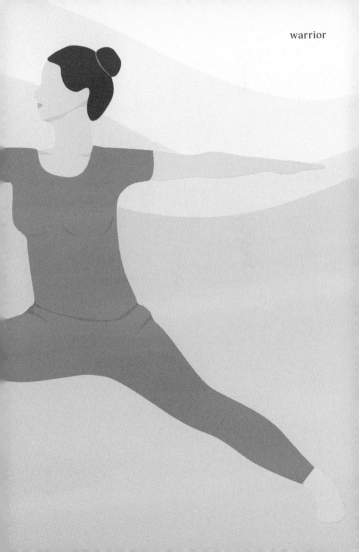

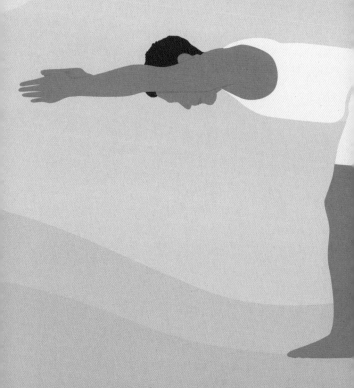

Warrior III

Virabhadrasana III

Think of your body creating the shape of a capital 'T' as you move into this pose; one leg is sent backward and arms together forward. Keep the leg and spine in line with each other, soft through the standing knee.

It can be wobbly but embrace that, as after all, we are all human! Find a point to focus on and breathe deeply.

Reverse Warrior

Viparita Virabhadrasana

Improve balance, core strength and mobility of the spine with Reverse Warrior.

Find a graceful bend in the top half of the body, the back hand slides down your back leg, top arm reaches over the head – think armpit to the sky. Legs should be strong and grounded in a wide Warrior II stance.

A pose to uplift your mood and boost your self-esteem.

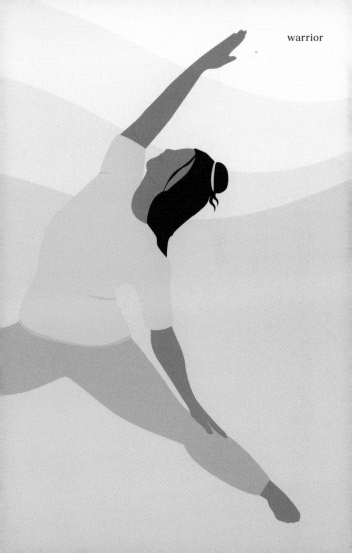

warrior

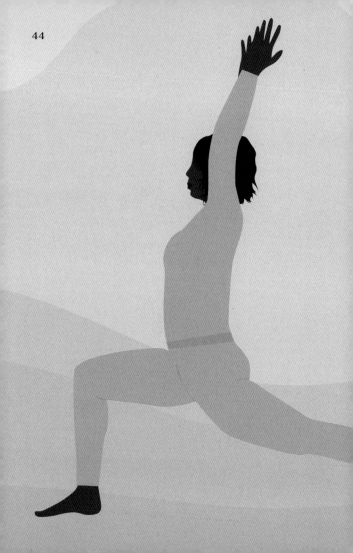

High Lunge

Ashta Chandrasana

A pose to find balance and stretch your feet, and to stabilize the muscles around the knee.

With both feet facing the front of your mat, bend the front leg to a right angle, opposite heel off the ground. Torso long and hands to sky, the gaze is forward and focused, bringing complete awareness to the entire body.

A pose to say to yourself 'I've got this'.

Straight Leg Triangle

Trikonasana

This pose can get confused with being a pose about the hamstrings, when actually it's a twist of the spine.

Starting in centre, feet wide, extend one hand to the sky and gently reach down the leg with the opposite hand. Guide your hips forward to find more of a twist in the upper body. Extend through the crown of the head, open the arms like wings, and breathe.

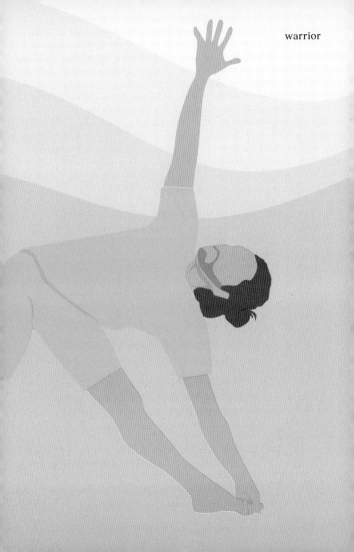

warrior

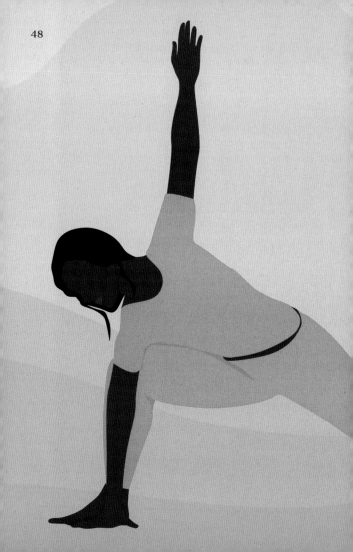

48

Extended Side Angle

Utthita Parsvakonasana

Feel the energy all the way through your body to your fingertips in this pose.

With your legs in Warrior II stance, place the same hand as the front leg on the inside of the front foot, then lift the opposite arm either up to the sky or over the head – gaze forward or up.

It's a pose with a strong force from underneath, drawing energy from the ground upwards to boost your energy and release fatigue.

Humble Warrior

Baddha Virabhadrasana

The Humble Warrior has many benefits:
a standing pose which opens the chest
and shoulders; a forward fold to draw the
attention inwards; and an inversion to
create more clarity and focus in the mind.

From Warrior II, reach your hands behind
and interlace the fingers, exhale and fold
the body forwards, hands moving above
your head as far as is comfortable. Allow
the head to relax as much as you can.

Make the pose humble
and surrender.

warrior

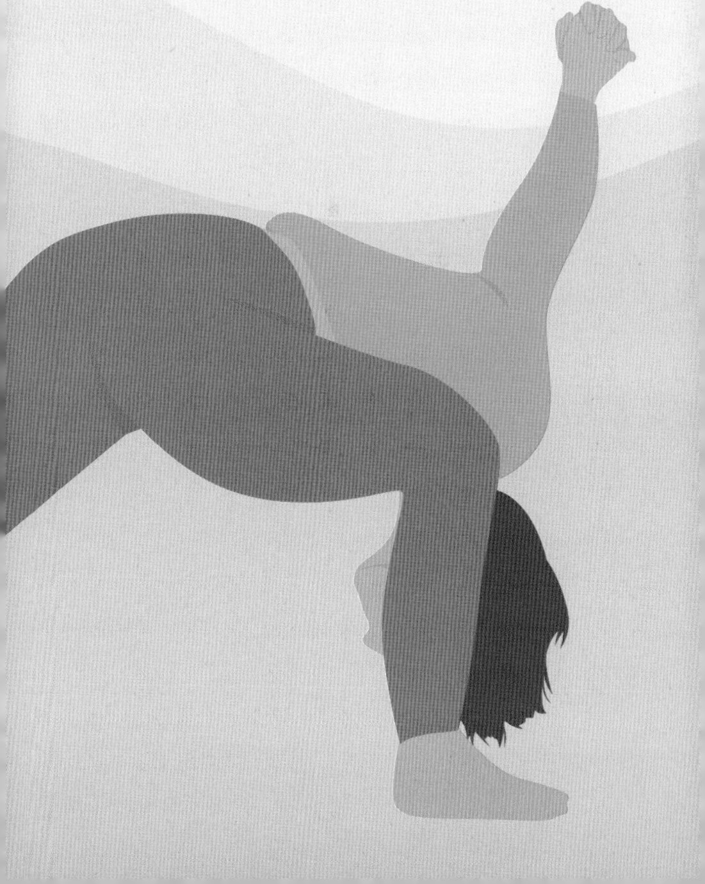

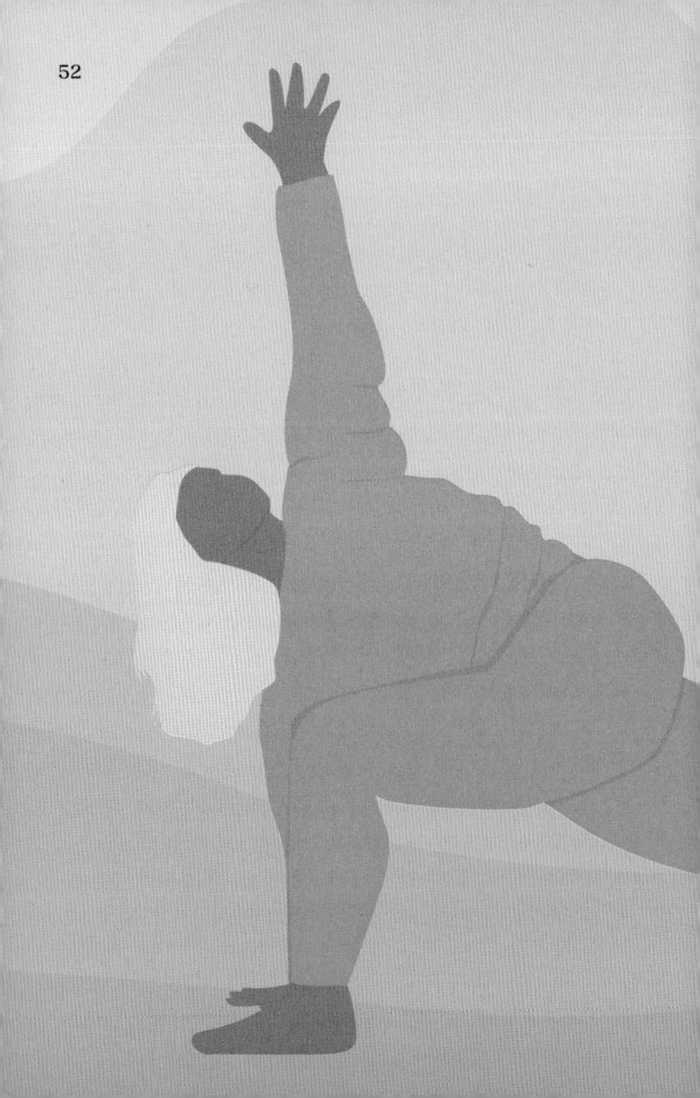

Twisted Lunge

Parivrtta Anjaneyasana

Twists always clear stagnant energy
from the spine, and this harmonizing
spine pose does just that.

Step one foot forward and place
the opposite hand to the ground.
Gently twist to open your side body
with the other hand to the sky.

Make sure your inner thighs are
engaged and that you are lifting
through the centre for this
twisting balance.

Standing Forward Fold

Uttanasana

A deep back body stretch, this Standing Forward Fold allows tension in the lower back to be released as you lower the body to the ground.

Inhale both arms up, stretch your fingertips to the sky, exhale and keep the knees soft as you fold the body forward. Allow the head to hang loosely.

Be soft, and enjoy this gentle inversion.

warrior

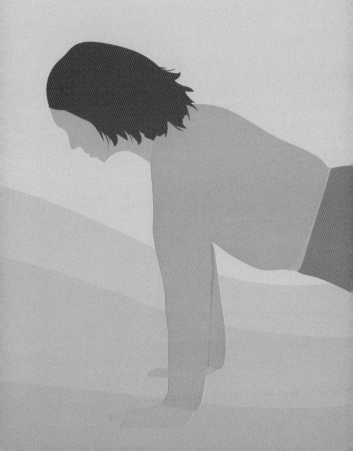

High Plank

Phalakasana

A pose to elevate your mood, this high plank position is a natural high even if it does feel like tough work whilst doing it!!

Keep your weight equal between the hands and the feet, holding strong through the core and head aligned with the spine.

Side Plank

Vasisthasana

A powerful arm and oblique pose, this can improve balance, concentration and focus. It can be intense on the arm and wrist, so modify to your needs if necessary.

You could drop the bottom knee to the floor for more support. Or if it feels very intense on your wrist, then come down onto your forearm instead, shoulder stacked over elbow.

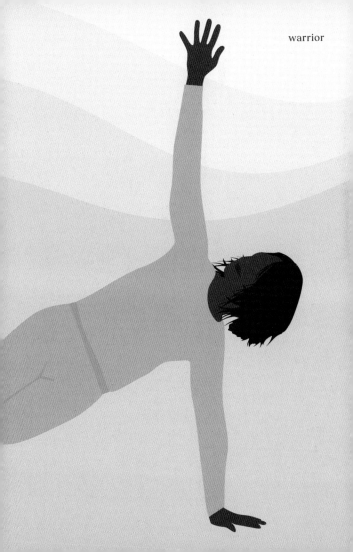

warrior

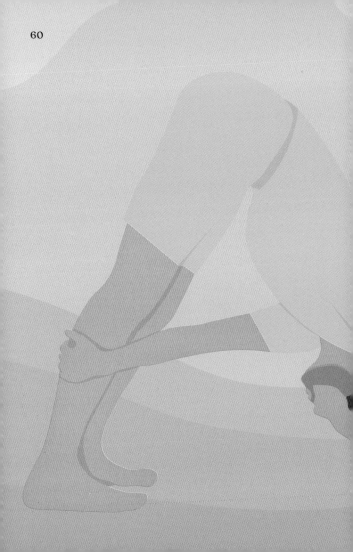

Twisted Downward Dog

Parivrtta Adho Mukha Svanasana

A relatively challenging variation on a classic pose, this twist of the torso massages and tones the internal organs, and offers a deeper lengthening of the hamstrings.

From Downward Dog, reach one hand under the body and across to the outside of the opposite foot, ankle or calf.

This is a whole body focus on balance and co-ordination.

Dolphin Pose

Ardha Pincha Mayurasana

If you are looking to build strength for inversions, then this is for you. Start in Downward Dog, look towards your hands and gently lower your elbows, one at a time, to the floor. Walk your feet forward, and keep looking forward, until you can't walk any further. Press your elbows firmly into the floor, and breathe!

This builds strength in the arms and shoulders, and flexibility in the upper back, hamstrings and calves. It's tough, but worth it.

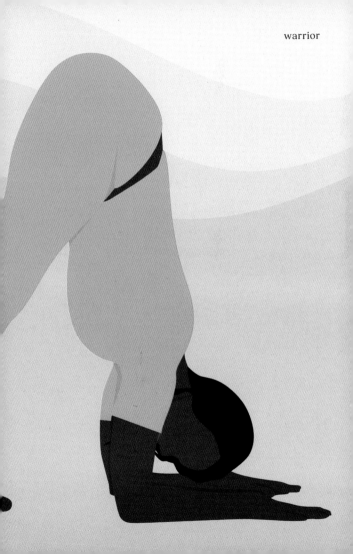

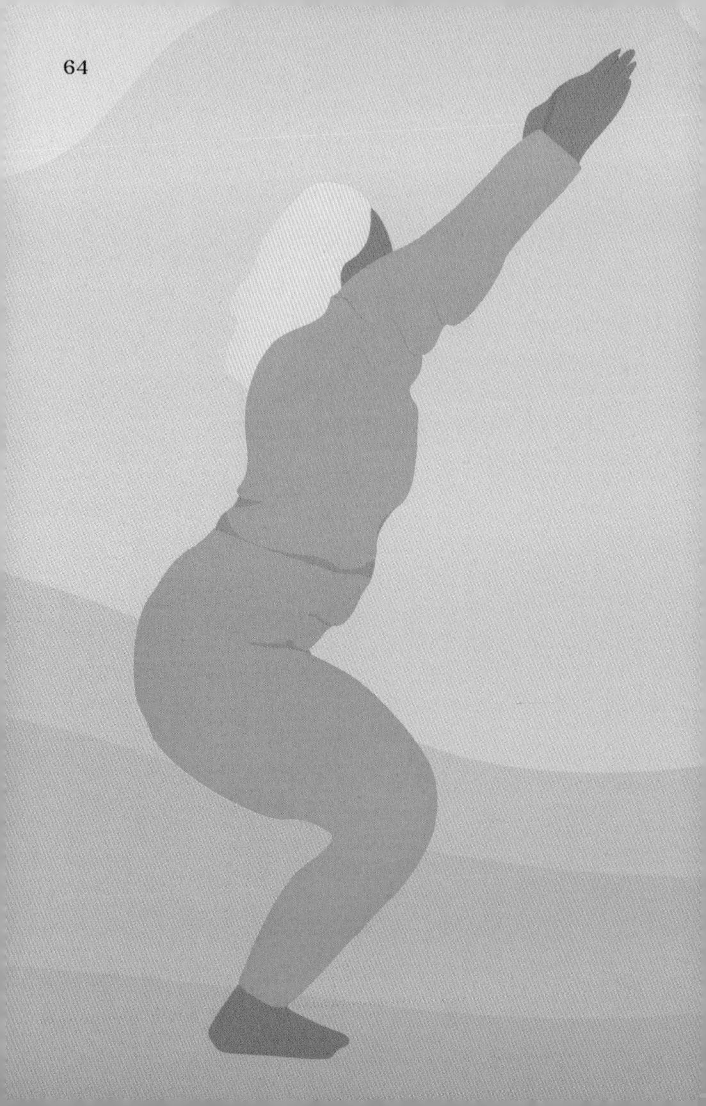

Chair Pose

Utkatasana

Bring the fire with this strong pose.

With both feet flat on the floor, inhale arms up to the sky, exhale and sink the hips down low as if you're sitting in a chair behind you.

Engage the whole back body, sit low, arms high and gain power and strength. This will stimulate the heart and be a challenge – sit as low as you can and breath long and deep.

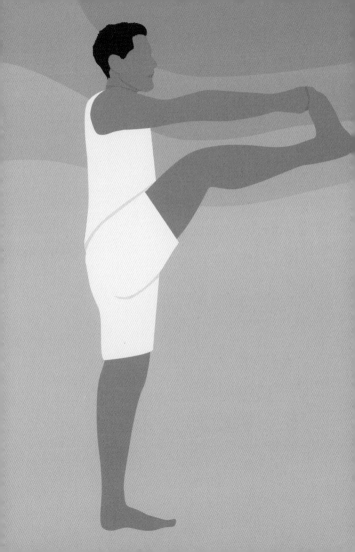

Tree Pose

Half Moon Pose

Standing Big Toe Stretch

Standing Splits

Standing Pigeon

Wide Leg Forward Fold

Goddess Pose

Eagle Pose

standing
balancing

Tree Pose

Vrikshasana

A joyful pose which calms the mind,
builds confidence and self-esteem,
and challenges your balance.

Grounding through the supporting
leg, press into the mat as you bring the
opposite foot up to meet the thigh or shin.

Find your balance, extend through the
spine, lift through the heart, find strength
in the core, and feel power all over.

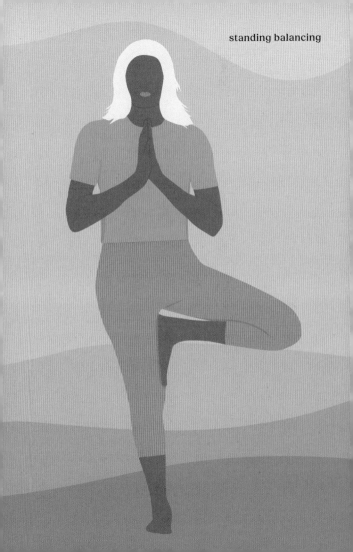

standing balancing

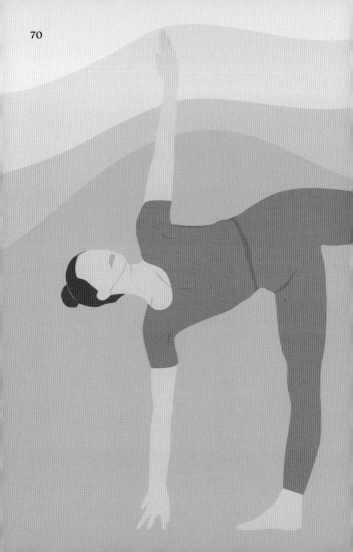

Half Moon Pose

Ardha Chandrasana

Imagine you are a big star with five points – arms, legs and head – extending away from the centre of the body.

Begin in a Warrior II stance, look forwards towards the floor, shift the weight into the front leg, and release the same hand as leg to the floor. Lift the back leg up to the sky. Feel the energy out through the fingertips and your toes.

Challenging for the body and mind, this can help alleviate back pain.

Standing Big Toe Stretch

Utthita Hasta Padangusthasana

This balancing pose opens the space between the toes and also stretches out the back of the legs. Lift from the hip, holding the toe with the hand on the same side. If you need to, keep the lifted knee bent or hold your knee instead of toe.

A pose to deepen your understanding of the distribution of weight between your feet and spine, to boost your energy and to fight fatigue.

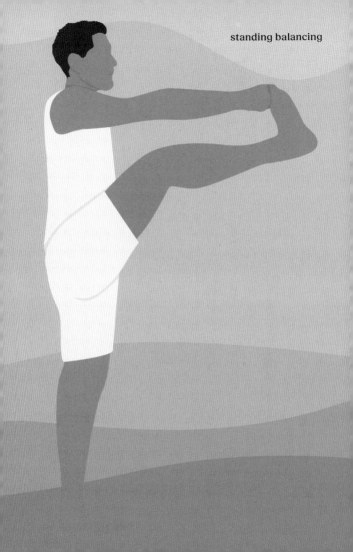

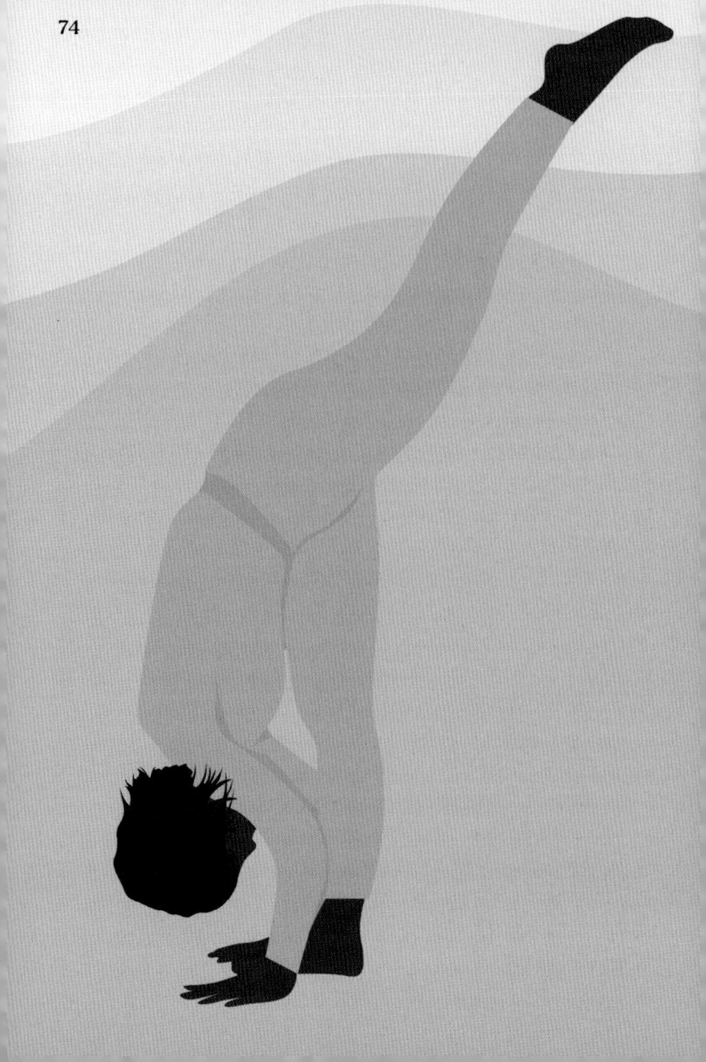

Standing Splits

Urdhva Prasarita Eka Padasana

The deepest of deep hamstring openers and a mild inversion that tests your balance.

Fold forward over the body, shift the weight into one foot, and on your next inhale lift the opposite leg behind you. Exhale and lift the leg higher – reaching for the sky, grounding down with the supporting leg. Slowly release back to a forward fold, and repeat on the opposite side.

Standing Pigeon

Tada Kapotasana

If you've been sitting down all day, this is a great end-of-the-day pose to loosen the hips. Bring one ankle to the opposite thigh, ground your foot, exhale and take a soft seat. Repeat on the other side.

A deep hip opening movement, it needs a strong balance and a totally focused mind. The sensation can be strong, so back off as you need. It also strengthens the knees and ankle joints, increasing mobility and range of motion.

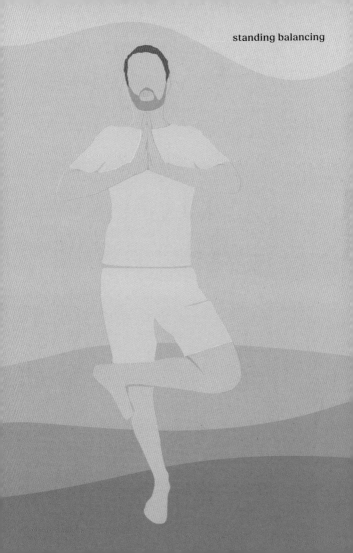

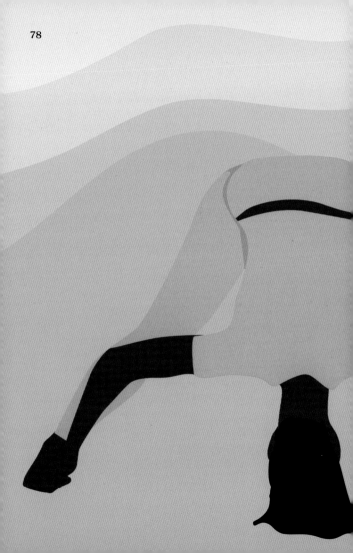

Wide Leg Forward Fold

Prasarita Padottanasana

A beautiful symmetrical shape that allows your pelvis and spine to stay neutral. Bend from your hip, and ground into the outside of the feet to keep the body stable.

This forward fold deeply activates the hamstrings, improves hip flexibility and also helps to strength the feet. It can be a great pose to decrease stress and anxiety – take a moment to turn inward.

Goddess Pose

Utkata Konasana

An empowering pose to connect to your inner strength, drawing energy from the ground upwards, allowing space and truth to expand through your heart.

With legs wide, turn the feet towards the corners of your mat. Exhale, bend the knees and lower your body, bringing the arms out bent at shoulder height.

A pose to step into when feeling foggy and needing clarity, confidence and self-belief.

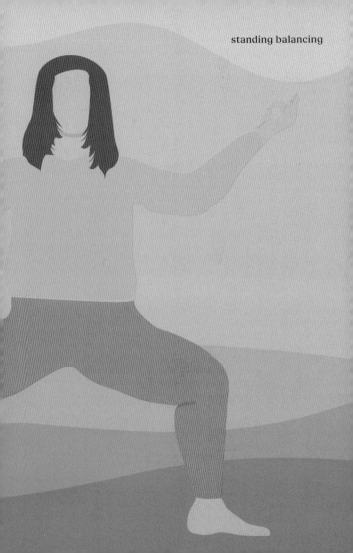

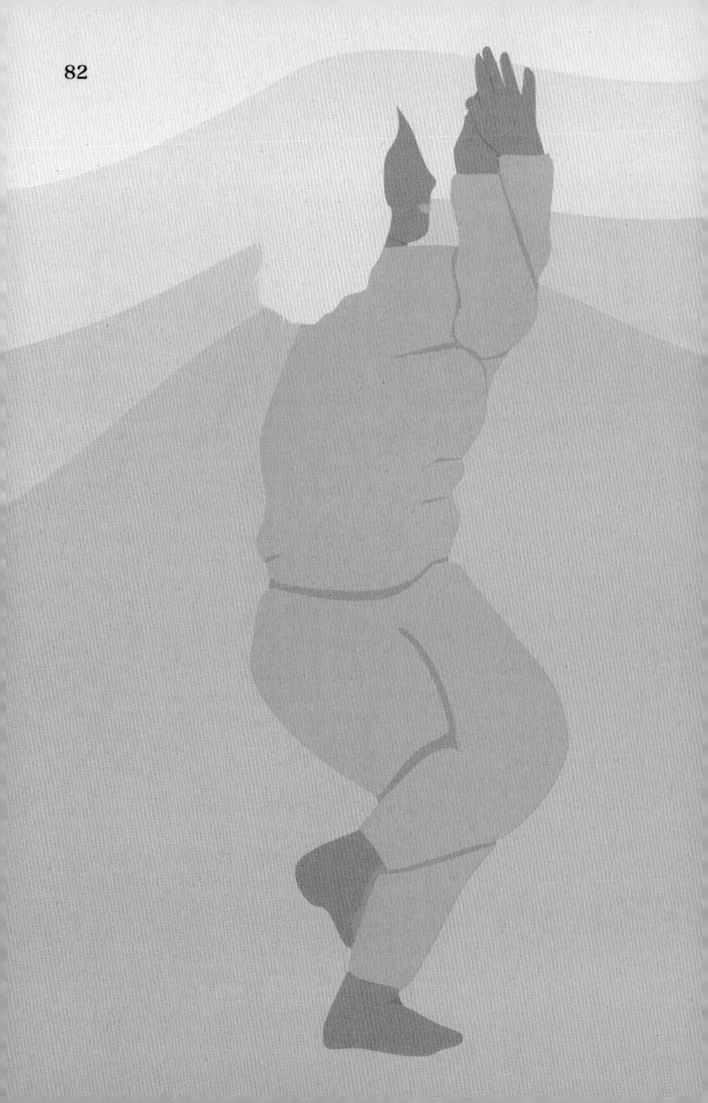

Eagle Pose

Garudasana

Take your time getting into this pose – find one spot to focus on to keep you balanced.

Cross one leg over the opposite thigh and curl the foot behind the calf, then wrap one arm around the other, squeezing both in towards the centre of the body.

This creates a deep hip opener and the arms wrapped together open the back of the lungs, increasing your ability to breathe deeper.

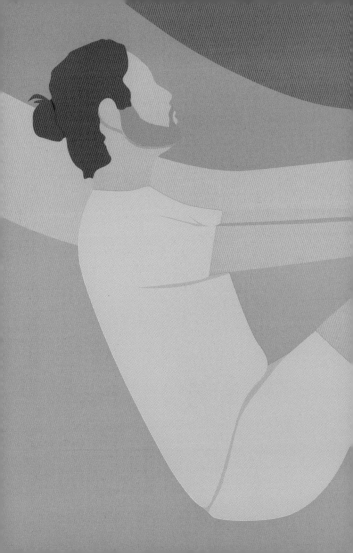

seated

Seated Twist

Ardha Matsyendrasana

A beautiful pose to cleanse and energize the whole spine, and a deeper variation of the Simple Seated Twist.

Sit tall to stimulate the digestive system, lengthen the body to better your posture, and try to make sure you turn the chin to really extend the twist all the way to the crown of your head.

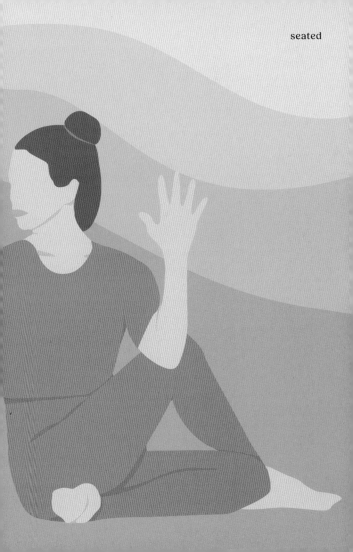

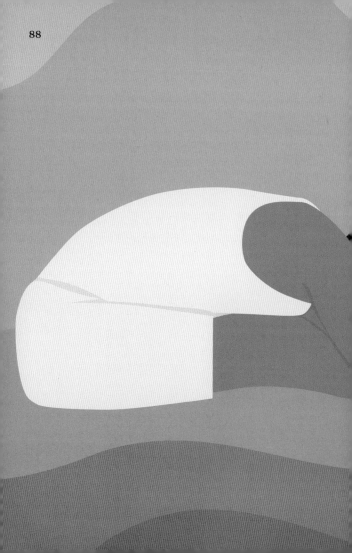

Seated Forward Bend

Paschimottanasana

A seated forward fold that will open the back of the legs, lower the spine, and release and stretch the shoulders.

Ease into the fold, and begin by holding the knees or calves if more comfortable. Keep the upper body soft, knees bent a little if you need, and breathe.

It's a very calming pose which allows you to draw your energy inwards, focusing the mind.

Reverse Plank

Purvottanasana

If you have been sat at a computer all day, then this pose is for you. It helps to release tension and open the chest and shoulders.

From a sitting position, slide the hands behind you, fingertips forward, and feet to the floor in front of you. Inhale and lift the hips high, grounding through the floor.

A strong pose to strengthen the wrists and arms, and find length all down the front side of the body.

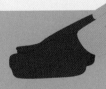

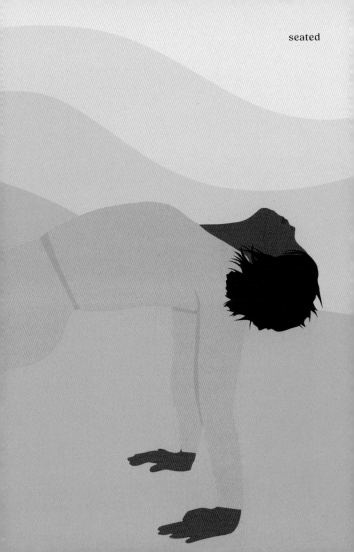

seated

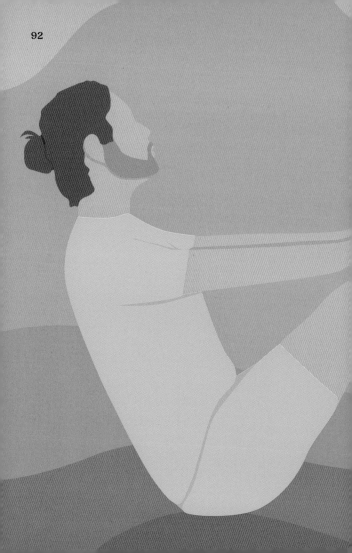

Boat Pose

Paripurna Navasana

This pose has many incredible benefits – it strengthens your inner core, hip flexors and adductor muscles, improves flexibility in the hamstrings and opens the chest.

From a seated position lean slightly backward and balance on your tailbone. Keep the back straight, lift the legs, shins parallel to the ground, then slowly straighten the knees and arms if possible.

A balancing pose which requires focus to increase your energy and confidence.

Dragon Pose

Utthan Pristhasana

Calling all runners, cyclists or those who sit down for large portions of the day – and that's a lot of us – this pose is for us all.

The hip flexors and quads get all the love here; go easy and gently, it's not called dragon for nothing! One leg comes forward, ankle under knee, opposite knee to the ground, and both hands to the ground on the inside of the front foot. You can stay on the hands, or perhaps come down on the elbows if that feels good for you.

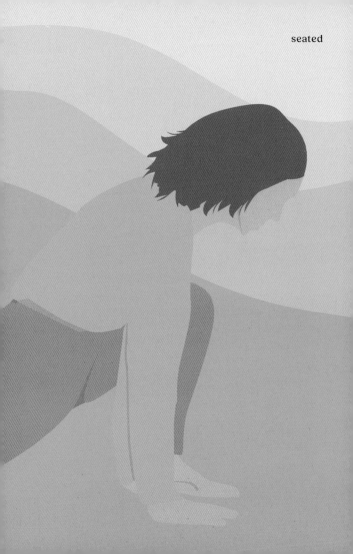

seated

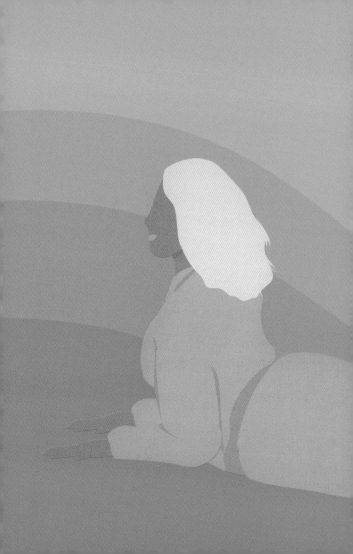

backbend

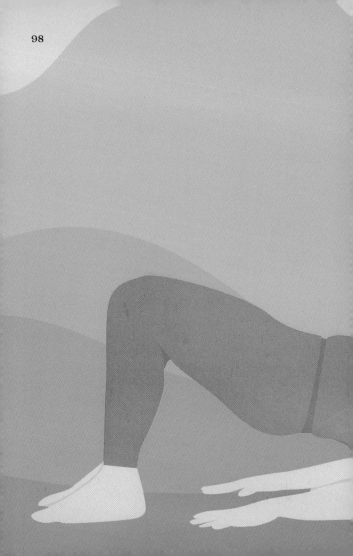

Bridge

Setu Bandha Sarvangasana

This inverted backbend allows you to feel the support of your upper body whist taking the pose.

Start on your back, feet hip width apart, hands by your hips. Lift the hips and press your feet into the floor, stretching and lengthening the whole front side of your body. This simultaneously strengthens the front and back of the body.

A pose to find stillness, alleviate stress and breathe.

Wild Thing

Camatkarasana

Super fun, dynamic and graceful, this strengthens the spine and stretches the front side of the legs. From Downward Dog raise one leg up to the sky and bend the knee to open your hip. From here you are going to flip your dog over. Move slowly – the leg that is in the air is going to stay bent and come to the earth, while the opposite leg is straight. It's a single hand backbend that enhances your whole overall body strength, channelling your inner dancer quality with the arms.

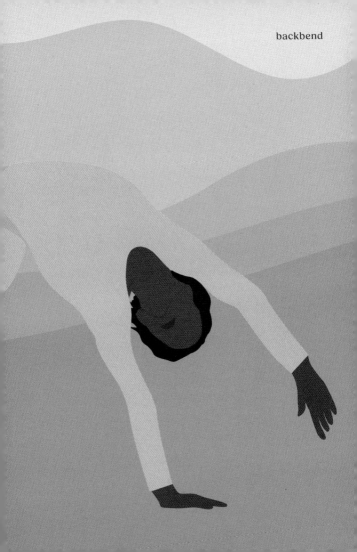

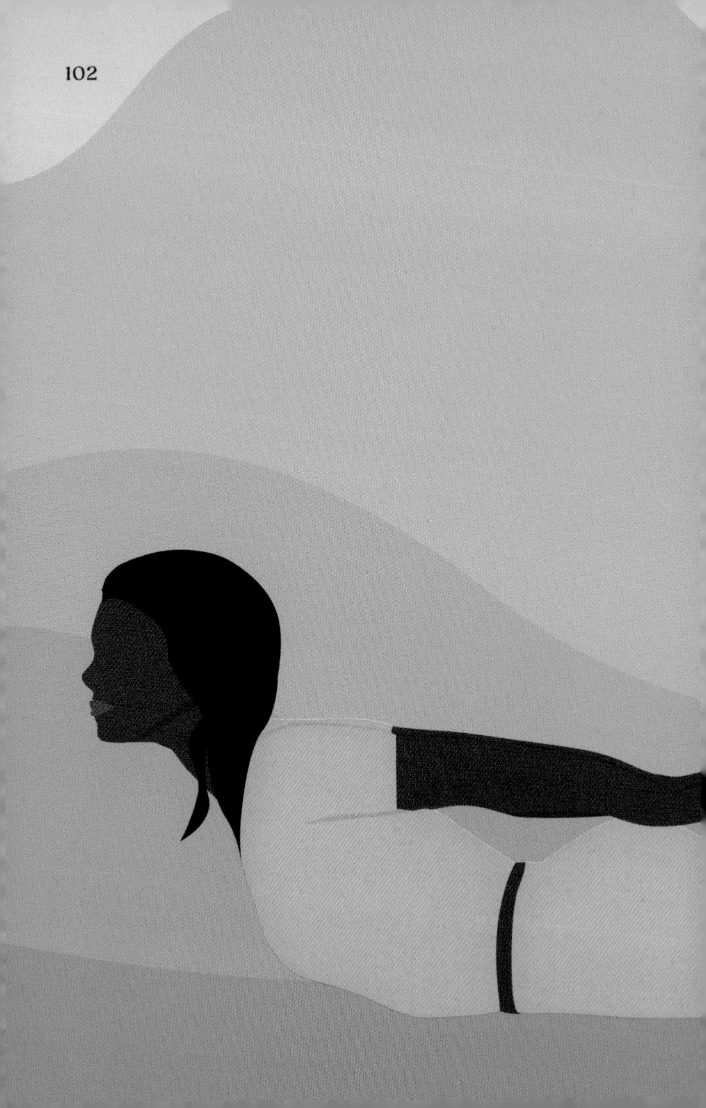

Locust Pose

Shalabasana

Draw up energy from the ground when coming into Locust. It is a strong strengthening pose for the back, but you will also feel the stretch and lengthening on your front side.

Roll the shoulders back and up away from the floor, gently raise the legs and arms behind your body.

Another great antidote for slouching spines and feeling low on energy.

Camel Pose

Ustrasana

An expansion of the upper body and elevation of the chest, this may take you a little out of your comfort zone. As always, remember to go as far as feels good for you.

Start kneeling on your shins, lean the body back and reach the hands back towards the heels. Take hold wherever feels comfortable. Heart reaches up, shoulders and chest open.

It's a natural booster of energy, a kick back to fatigue and the perfect afternoon pick me up.

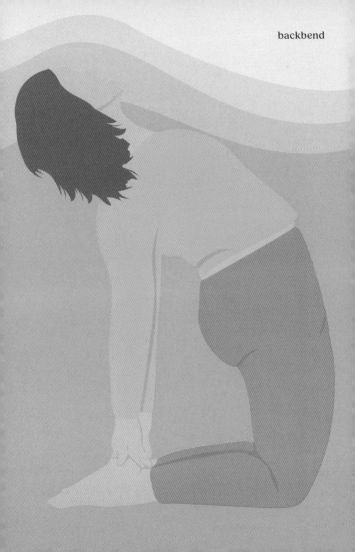

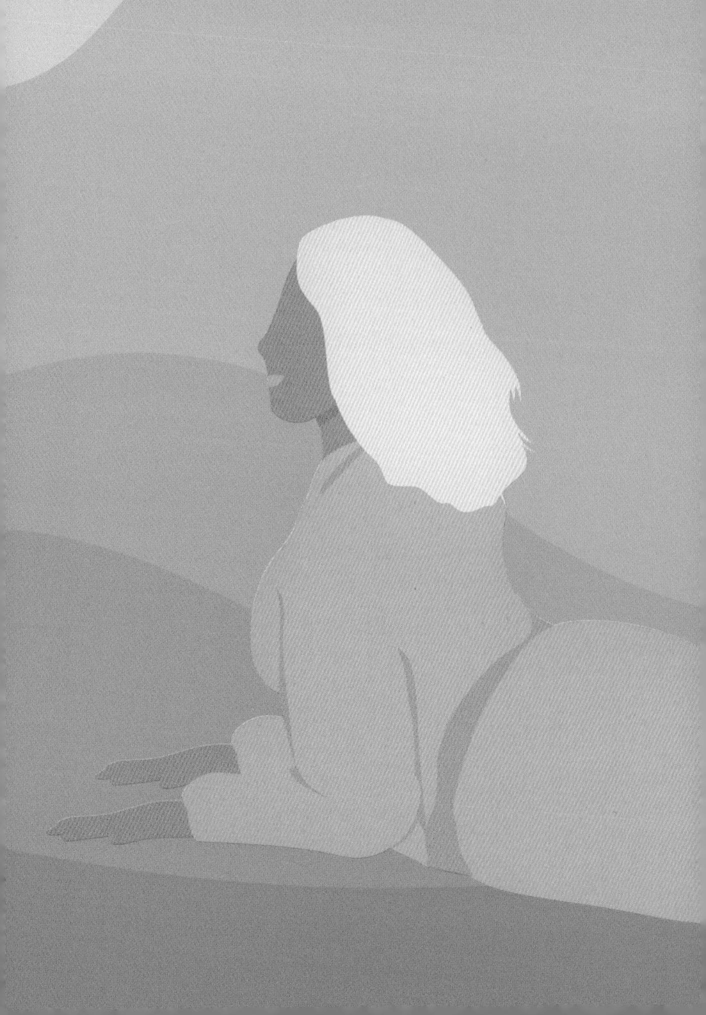

Sphinx Pose

Salamba Bhujangasana

Just like the mythical creatures that stand in Egypt, this shape has an air of elegance and poise. A soft back bend with the support of your arms, it invigorates the body and soothes the nervous system.

From lying front down, draw your elbows back in line with the shoulders and slowly rise up, open the heart and feel the stretch through the back body.

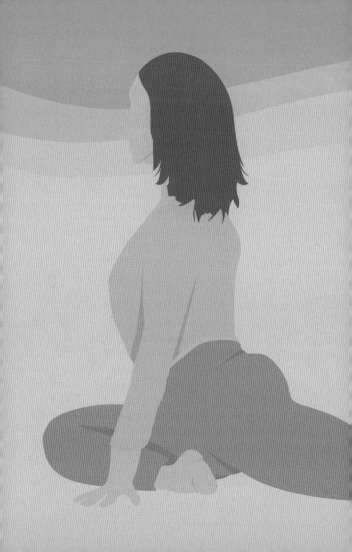

Reclined Butterfly
Happy Baby
Supine Twist
Pigeon Pose
Shoulder Stand
Head Stand
Corpse Pose

closing
poses

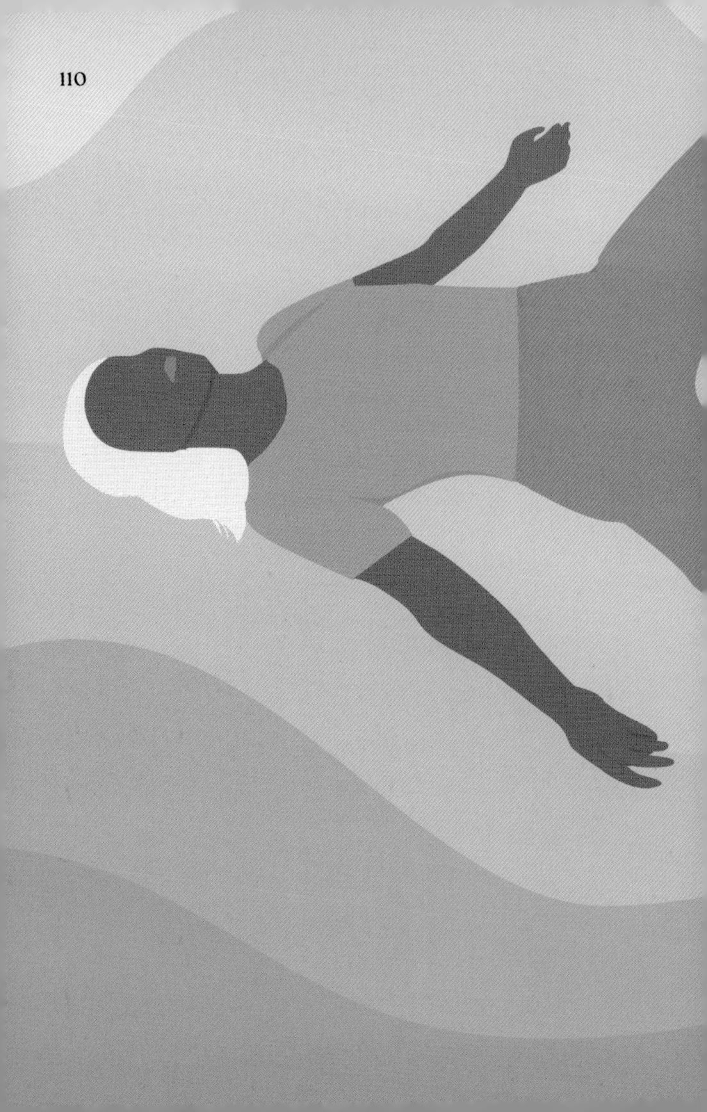

Reclined Butterfly

Supta Baddha Konasana

This pose is the ultimate surrender pose. From a seated position, bring the soles of the feet together with your knees out to the side. Gently recline the upper body back onto the floor. If it feels too intense on the inner thighs, slide the feet further away from the groin. Palms facing the sky, allow this simple gesture of open hands to soften your whole body and mind.

This pose is known to alleviate upper and lower back pain and can ease stress.

Happy Baby

Ananda Balasana

Hello inner thighs! The groin is an area of sensitivity, so follow the lead of your body when you come into this pose. Inhale, both feet to the sky, holding onto the outside of the feet or ankles – gently encourage the knees to the earth, no pulling!

This pose should bring you all the joy, so allow yourself to feel it. It offers a release in the lower back, and a little rock from side to side can feel amazing. Stay close to the earth, keeping grounded and balanced.

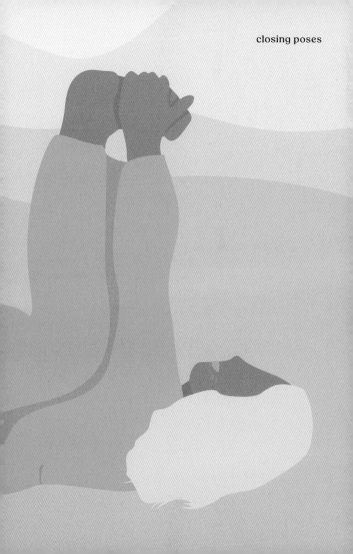

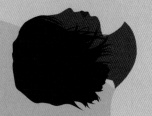

Supine Twist

Supta Matsyendrasana

The most delicious twist to balance and harmonize the body after your practice.

On your back, simply allow your knee to fall to the opposite side and look the other way. Your arms can be however you like, whatever feels comfortable.

This twist enables more movement and flexibility in your spine, and also can aid with digestion.

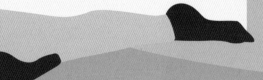

Pigeon Pose

Eka Pada Rajakapotasana

Feel the deep, grounding and strong stretching sensations in this pose. A shape to stay in for a long time if you can.

From Downward Dog, bring one foot forward and place the knee on the ground in front of the body. Lower yourself down and feel the stretch through the hips.

Mobility and flexibility of the hips are targeted, and you may also feel a stretch in the groin area. It's like medicine for the joints.

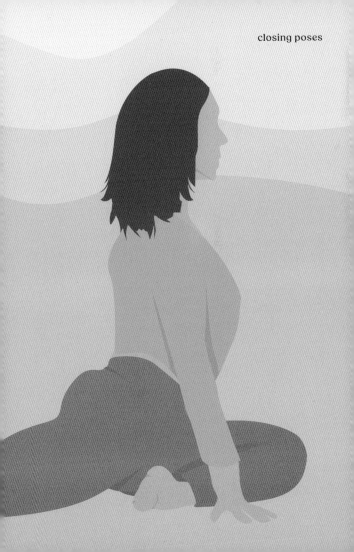

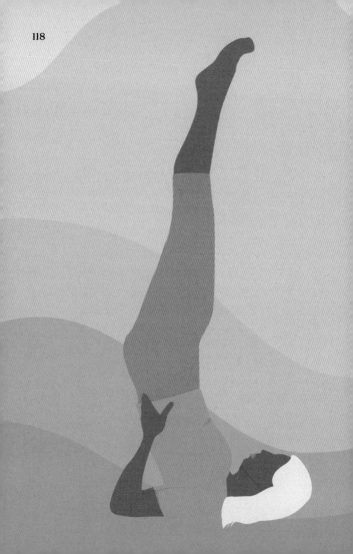

Shoulder Stand

Sarvangasana

Give your legs a moment to rest from being on the ground all the time.

The lift and hold needed for this pose creates a lot of core and upper body strength. Allow the feet to come over your head to the sky, supporting the lower back with your hands, elbows bent and grounded.

An inversion to see the world and your feet from a different perspective!

Head Stand

Salamba Sirsasana

Known as the king of asanas, this pose
may feel like the biggest journey
to achieve.

Start in Child's Pose. Interlace the
hands on the floor, then place the top
of your head down, cradled by your
hands. Each time you practice go
a little further – start by lifting the
knees, then walking the feet forward,
then (without jumping) lifting each
knee to your chest. This is not a pose
to rush. It will come to you when your
body and mind are strong enough,
and you feel comfortable and ready.

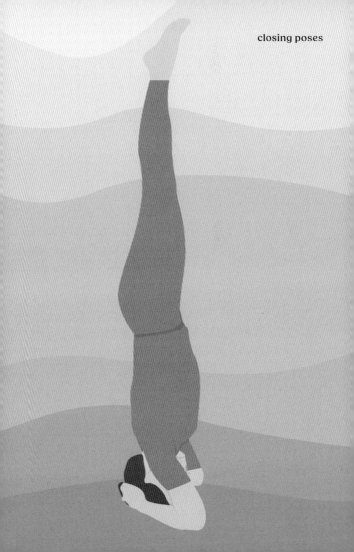

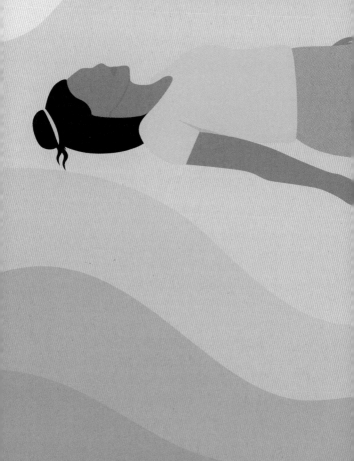

Corpse Pose

Savasana

The final resting pose to all yoga practices and definitely not one that should ever be missed out.

Allowing the body to be still after moving gives your muscles a chance to remember all the instructions and positions it has been placed in, and muscle memory is so powerful.

There is no greater power than rest, remember that rest is not a luxury but a necessity for us to thrive.

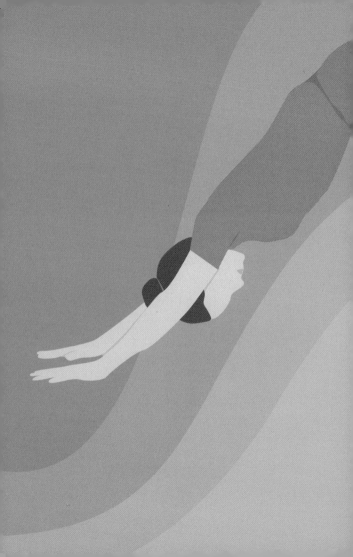

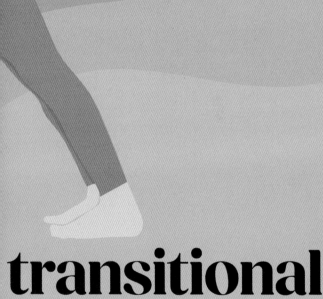

transitional

Downward Dog

Upward Dog

Low Plank

Downward Dog

Adho Mukha Svanasana

The intention of this pose is to find length in the back of the body. Press the hands down into your mat to allow the energy from below to empower you.

From all fours tuck your toes under and gently lift your hips to the sky. Keep the heels raised if it feels more comfortable.

Breathe deeply in this soft inversion, and allow yourself to see the world from a different perspective.

Upward Dog

Urdhva Mukha Svanasana

An amazing antidote to your 'office chair slump'. Feel a deep chest and shoulder opening, while also strengthening the spine, arms and wrist.

Lie on your front, bring your hands in line with your shoulders and gently lift up. Remember to keep your legs engaged to spread the weight, and think forwards and upwards for this posture-improving pose.

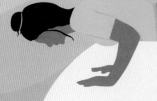

Low Plank

Chaturanga Dandasana

This pose can feel hard, especially at the beginning of your yoga journey, but remember that you can always modify it by placing the knees on the floor.

It's a strong pose to strengthen your whole body; it is great for your spine and improving posture, as well as stimulating and energizing the mind.